SURVIVING UTERINE CANCER

I0446783

**Beginners Comprehensive
Approach To Combating &
Managing Uterine Cancer
Outbreak Effectively**

Nuel Nenji

Table of Contents

Introductory

Uterine cancer, also known as endometrial cancer, is a form of cancer that begins in the endometrium, the uterine lining. The uterus is a pear-shaped organ in the pelvis of a woman's reproductive system where the embryo develops during pregnancy.

Typically, uterine cancer originates when endometrial cells undergo genetic mutations that cause them to proliferate uncontrollably. Within the uterus, these abnormal cells can create a mass or tumor. Over time, if left untreated, uterine cancer can spread to nearby tissues and, in advanced phases, to distant organs through a process called metastasis.

Uterine cancer is the most prevalent type of gynecologic cancer in women, and it predominantly affects postmenopausal women, though it can affect women of any age.

Certain risk factors can increase a person's likelihood of developing uterine cancer, although its precise cause is not always clear. Among these risk factors are:

• Imbalance of Hormones: An excess of estrogen relative to progesterone can increase the risk of uterine cancer. This hormonal imbalance can be caused by polycystic ovary syndrome (PCOS) and estrogen replacement therapy without progestin.

• Age: The risk of uterine cancer increases with age, with postmenopausal women being the most susceptible.

• Being overweight or obese increases the likelihood of developing uterine cancer.

• Endometrial Hyperplasia: This condition is characterized by the abnormal proliferation of endometrial cells and is in some cases considered a precursor to uterine cancer.

• A family history of uterine cancer or certain inherited disorders, such as Lynch syndrome, may increase the risk.

• Women with diabetes have an increased risk of developing uterine cancer.

• This medication, which is commonly used to treat breast cancer, has been linked to an increased risk of developing uterine cancer.

Abnormal vaginal bleeding, particularly postmenopausal bleeding, is the most common symptom of uterine cancer. Other symptoms may include pelvic pain, discomfort during sexual activity, and a uterus that is enlarged.

Detection and diagnosis at an early stage are essential for the successful treatment of uterine cancer. Treatment options typically entail surgery to remove the uterus (hysterectomy) and may also include radiation therapy, chemotherapy, and hormone therapy, depending on the stage and characteristics of the cancer.

It is important for individuals, particularly those with risk factors, to be aware of the symptoms of uterine cancer and to seek medical attention immediately if they experience such symptoms.

In addition to regular gynecological examinations and discussions with a healthcare provider about risk factors and preventive measures, regular gynecological examinations and discussions about risk factors and preventive measures can be beneficial in reducing the risk of uterine cancer.

CHAPTER ONE
Types And Causes Of Uterine Cancer

Uterine cancer, also known as endometrial cancer, originates predominantly in the endometrium, the uterine lining. However, there are several distinct varieties of uterine cancer, each with its own characteristics. The two primary types of uterine cancer are:

1. Type I Endometrioid Carcinoma:

• Endometrioid carcinoma is the most prevalent form of uterine cancer, and it is frequently linked to hormonal imbalances, specifically an excess of estrogen relative to progesterone.

Endometrioid carcinoma risk is increased by conditions that result in protracted estrogen exposure, such as obesity, estrogen replacement therapy without progestin, and polycystic ovary syndrome (PCOS).

• This form of uterine cancer tends to grow slowly and is frequently diagnosed at an earlier stage. It typically affects perimenopausal and menopausal women.

2. Type II Non-Endometrioid Carcinoma:

• Non-endometrioid carcinomas are less common than endometrioid carcinomas, but tend to be more aggressive. They are not strongly linked to estrogen and progesterone imbalances and are significantly less influenced by hormonal factors.

• This category comprises several subtypes, including serous carcinoma and clear cell carcinoma. Non-endometrioid carcinomas are typically diagnosed at a later stage and necessitate a more aggressive treatment strategy.

In addition to these two primary varieties of uterine cancer, there are other rare types, including:

3. Cancer of the uterus:

• Causes: Uterine sarcomas are uncommon and originate from the uterine muscle or connective tissue, not the endometrium. Some genetic factors and prior pelvic radiation therapy may be linked to an increased risk, but the precise causes are not well understood.

• Uterine sarcomas are typically more aggressive than endometrial carcinomas, necessitating distinct treatment strategies.

Noting that the specific causes of uterine cancer are not always clear-cut, and that the development of this cancer frequently involves a combination of genetic, hormonal, and environmental factors, is essential. As mentioned previously, certain risk factors can increase the likelihood of developing uterine cancer. These consist of:

• Hormonal imbalances, specifically estrogen excess.

• Aging, with the majority of cases affecting postmenopausal women.

• Morbid obesity.

• A history of uterine or related malignancies in the family.

• Specific genetic syndromes, including Lynch syndrome.

• Diabetes mellitus.

• Prior treatment with tamoxifen for breast cancer.

Understanding the various types of uterine cancer and the risk factors associated with each type is essential for early detection and effective treatment. Regular gynecological check-ups and discussions with healthcare providers can help assess individual risk and determine appropriate preventive measures and screenings.

Menstruation And Uterine Alterations

The menstrual cycle a complex, orchestrated process that predominantly involves the uterus and ovaries in the female reproductive system. It is controlled by a series of hormonal fluctuations and functions to prepare the body for potential pregnancy.

In response to these hormonal fluctuations, the uterus endures various changes throughout the menstrual cycle.

Here is a summary of the menstrual cycle and associated uterine changes:

1. Phase menstruale (days 1-5):

• Hormonal Alterations: At the beginning of the menstrual cycle, estrogen and progesterone levels are low.

• Uterine Changes: During this phase, the endometrium from the previous cycle is released through the vagina, causing menstruation.

2. Folicular Phase (1-13 days):

• The pituitary gland secretes follicle-stimulating hormone (FSH), which stimulates the ovaries to produce estrogen. A dominant ovarian follicle harboring an egg (ovum) develops when estrogen levels rise.

• Uterine Changes: In response to rising estrogen levels, the endometrium begins to regenerate and thicken, preparing a nourishing environment for a potential embryo.

3. Ovulation (approximately Day 14):

• Hormonal Alterations: An increase in luteinizing hormone (LH) causes the mature egg to be released from the ovarian follicle.

• Uterine Alterations: The endometrium continues to thicken, and glands in the uterine lining begin secreting substances that can support fertilization and implantation.

4. Luteal Phase (15-28 days):

• Hormonal Changes: Following ovulation, the ovarian follicle transforms into the corpus luteum, a structure that produces progesterone. The levels of progesterone rise while estrogen levels remain elevated.

• Uterine Changes: Under the influence of estrogen and progesterone, the uterine lining continues to thicken, creating an optimal environment for embryo implantation. The endometrium's blood vessels become more prominent, resulting in an abundant blood supply.

5. Menstruation (If Pregnancy Does Not Occur):

• Hormonal Changes: In the absence of fertilization, the corpus luteum degenerates, resulting in a decrease in estrogen and progesterone levels.

• Uterine Alterations: The decrease in hormone levels causes the discharge of the thickened uterine lining, which results in menstruation and the beginning of a new menstrual cycle.

If conception occurs, the fertilized egg typically implants into the thickened uterine lining, and the hormonal environment supports the growth and development of the embryo and later the fetus.

The menstrual cycle is an essential component of the female reproductive system, and the uterine alterations that occur during this cycle are essential for fertility and the possibility of conception. Understanding these hormonal and uterine alterations is crucial to reproductive health management and family planning.

CHAPTER TWO
Indications And Symptoms

Signs and symptoms of various medical conditions can vary considerably based on the nature and severity of the condition. Below is a list of prevalent signs and symptoms that may indicate a variety of health conditions.

Noting that these are general symptoms and that experiencing one or more does not necessarily indicate a specific diagnosis is essential. It is essential to consult a healthcare professional for a thorough evaluation and diagnosis if you are experiencing concerning symptoms.

- A fever typically indicates an infection or inflammatory response.

- Fatigue: Numerous underlying conditions, including anemia, chronic diseases, and sleep disorders, can cause persistent fatigue or a lack of energy.

- Pain can be caused by injuries, infections, inflammation, or chronic conditions and can manifest in various regions of the body.

- Headaches can be caused by a variety of factors, including tension, migraines, sinus problems, and more severe conditions such as intracranial pressure.

• Nausea and vomiting can be caused by gastrointestinal disorders, infections, pregnancy, motion sickness, or medication adverse effects.

• A persistent wheeze may be the result of respiratory infections, allergies, asthma, or other lung disorders.

• Breathing Difficulties: Breathing difficulties may indicate respiratory or cardiac issues, allergies, or anxiety.

• Chest Pain: Chest pain is a symptom of cardiac problems (angina or heart attack), gastrointestinal issues, and musculoskeletal disorders.

• Unexplained Weight Loss: Sudden or unexplained weight loss may indicate a number of underlying health conditions, such as metabolic disorders, cancer, or thyroid issues.

• Changes in Bowel Habits: Persistent diarrhea, constipation, blood in stools, and alterations in stool appearance may indicate gastrointestinal issues or colon cancer.

• Men who urinate frequently may have urinary tract infections, diabetes, or prostate problems.

• Vision Alterations: Blurred vision, double vision, and vision loss may be caused by eye conditions, migraines, or neurological disorders.

• Dermatologist evaluation is required for skin symptoms such as rashes, irritation, redness, or changes in moles.

• Joint Pain is a symptom of arthritis, autoimmune diseases, and trauma.

• Mood Swings: Mood swings, depression, anxiety, and behavioral alterations may be caused by mental health conditions, stress, or underlying medical conditions.

• Neurological Symptoms: Numbness, tingle, weakness, or coordination issues may indicate neurological disorders or nerve-related problems.

• The swelling of the extremities or other regions of the body may be caused by fluid retention, heart disease, kidney disease, or injury.

• Frequent infections may be indicative of a compromised immune system or underlying medical conditions.

• Gastrointestinal Symptoms: Symptoms such as bloating, abdominal pain, heartburn, or dyspepsia can be related to gastrointestinal disorders like gastritis, irritable bowel syndrome

(IBS), or gastroesophageal reflux disease (GERD).

• Changes in menstrual patterns, such as heavy bleeding, irregular periods, or delayed periods, may be caused by gynecological disorders or hormonal imbalances.

These are merely some of the prevalent signs and symptoms that people may experience when dealing with a variety of health problems. It is essential to keep in mind that symptoms can vary widely, and a comprehensive medical evaluation is necessary to determine the underlying cause and appropriate treatment. If you or a loved one are experiencing persistent or severe symptoms, it is advisable to seek medical attention as soon as possible.

The diagnosis and staging of a medical condition, especially cancer, are crucial stages in determining the disease's severity, its characteristics, and the optimal treatment.

Below, I will describe the general process of diagnosis and staging, using cancer as an illustration.

Clinical diagnosis:

• Medical History and Physical Examination: The first stage typically consists of a thorough medical history interview and a physical examination by a healthcare professional. During this procedure, the symptoms, risk factors, and pertinent medical history of the patient are discussed.

• Blood tests and other laboratory tests, such as complete blood count (CBC), blood chemistry, and tumor markers, may be used to evaluate various parameters. These tests can provide valuable information regarding the patient's overall health and the prevalence of specific markers associated with a variety of diseases.

• Imaging Studies: X-rays, computed tomography (CT) scans, magnetic resonance imaging (MRI), ultrasound, and positron emission tomography

(PET) scans may be utilized to visualize internal structures and detect abnormalities.

These images aid in the detection of tumors, evaluation of their size and location, and determination of whether the cancer has migrated to other areas of the body.

• A biopsy may be performed if imaging reveals suspicious findings or if there are clinical indications. A biopsy entails the removal of a small tissue or cell sample from the affected area, which is then examined by a pathologist under a microscope to confirm the presence of cancer and determine its type and grade.

• Endoscopy: When cancer is suspected in the digestive tract or other internal organs, endoscopy may be conducted. This procedure permits direct visualization of the interior of organs and the collection of biopsied tissue samples.

Setting up:

The process of determining the extent and dissemination of cancer in the body is known as staging. Staging is vital because it guides treatment decisions and aids in prognosis prediction. The TNM system (Tumor, Node, and Metastasis) and numerical stage classifications are common staging systems for cancer.

• This component of the staging system evaluates the size and scope of the primary tumor. Typically, T categories span from 0 (in situ, confined to the organ of origin) to higher numbers, which indicate tumors that are larger and more invasive.

• N (Node): N categories indicate the involvement of nearby lymph nodes. Lymph nodes are small, bean-shaped structures that filter lymphatic fluid and can function as a conduit for the spread of malignancy. the lymph node involvement.

• M denotes whether the cancer has spread to distant organs or tissues. M0 indicates that there are no distant metastases, while M1 indicates that there are distant metastases.

• When the T, N, and M categories are combined, the overall cancer stage is determined. The stages are frequently designated with Roman numerals (e.g., Stage I, Stage II) and may include subcategories (e.g., Stage IIA, Stage IIB) to provide additional information about the disease's progression.

The cancer's stage is crucial in determining the treatment strategy. Early-stage malignancies are typically treated with localized therapies (surgery or radiation therapy), whereas advanced-stage cancers may require more aggressive treatments, including chemotherapy, targeted therapy, immunotherapy, or a combination of these approaches.

Diagnosis and staging of medical conditions necessitate a multidisciplinary approach involving input from oncologists, radiologists, pathologists, and surgeons, among others. Accurate diagnosis and staging are essential for customizing the most effective and appropriate treatment plan for each patient.

The Significance Of Early Diagnosis

The significance of early detection of medical conditions, particularly cancer and chronic diseases, cannot be overstated.

• Improved Treatment Outcomes: Early disease detection frequently results in more effective treatment options and improved overall treatment outcomes. Many cancers, for instance, are more curable if detected at an early, localized stage, before they have spread to other regions of the body.

• Early-stage diseases may necessitate less aggressive and invasive treatments than advanced-stage diseases. This can result in fewer adverse effects and an improvement in patients' quality of life.

• Early detection can lead to less expensive treatments and a lighter burden on healthcare systems, resulting in lower healthcare costs. Treatments for diseases in their advanced stages are frequently more extensive and costly.

• Prolonged Survival: Early detection can result in increased patient survival rates. Many diseases, including cancer, have substantially higher survival rates if diagnosed and treated in their early stages.

• Preservation of Organ Function: Detecting and treating diseases early may help preserve the function of affected organs. For instance, early treatment of kidney disease or diabetes can prevent kidney and other vital organ injury.

• Early detection can prevent or reduce the risk of complications associated with certain diseases. For instance, early intervention in diabetes can aid in the prevention of complications such as kidney failure, blindness, and cardiovascular disease.

• Improved Quality of Life Detection at an early stage can result in a higher quality of life for patients. Early disease management and treatment can prevent symptoms from aggravating and interfering with daily activities.

• Screening and Preventive Measures: Regular screenings and preventive measures, such as immunizations and adjustments in lifestyle, can reduce the risk of developing certain diseases in the first place.

• Psychological Benefits: Early disease diagnosis can reduce the anxiety associated with uncertainty. It enables patients and their healthcare providers to address the condition proactively, thereby reducing stress and anxiety.

• Impact on Public Health Population-level early detection and prevention efforts can have a significant impact on public health. Early disease detection can help control outbreaks, reduce healthcare costs, and enhance the overall health of a community.

It's crucial to note that the specific benefits of early detection may vary depending on the disease and individual circumstances. Not all diseases have effective methods for early detection, and not everyone has access to regular screenings or healthcare.

Nevertheless, the general principle maintains that identifying and treating diseases in their earliest stages can have a significant impact on patient outcomes and public health as a whole. Regular medical examinations, screenings, and a healthy lifestyle can aid in early detection and improved health outcomes

CHAPTER THREE
Therapeutic Options

Depending on the specific condition, its stage or severity, as well as the patient's health status and preferences, treatment options for medical conditions can vary considerably. I will now provide an overview of prevalent treatment options that may be considered for a variety of medical conditions.

1. Medical treatments:

• Prescription Drugs: Antibiotics for infections, insulin for diabetes, and chemotherapy for cancer are examples of prescription medications that can be used to treat a variety of medical conditions.

• Nonprescription medications, such as pain relievers, antacids, and allergy medications, can mitigate the symptoms of specific conditions.

2. Surgical Techniques:

• Surgical Procedures: Surgery can be used to treat a variety of conditions, including the removal of malignancies and the repair of injuries, as well as organ transplantations and weight loss surgeries.

• Minimally Invasive Surgery: Techniques such as laparoscopy and robotic surgery involve smaller incisions and shorter recuperation times than conventional open surgery.

3. Radiation Treatment:

• Radiation therapy employs high-energy radiation beams to target and kill cancer cells. It is commonly used to treat a variety of malignancies.

4. Cancer chemotherapy:

• Chemotherapy utilizes drugs to kill or halt the development of cancer cells. It can be administered alone or in conjunction with other therapies, such as radiation or surgery.

5. Vaccine therapy:

• Immunotherapy is a form of cancer treatment that stimulates the patient's immune system to recognize cancer cells and attack them. Certain varieties of cancer have been successfully treated with this technique.

6. Targeted Treatment:

• In targeted therapy, specific molecules or proteins implicated in cancer growth are targeted by drugs. Specific forms of cancer are treated with minimal effect on healthy cells.

7. Hormone Replacement:

• Hormone therapy is commonly employed in the treatment of hormone-sensitive cancers such as breast and prostate cancer in order to inhibit or alter hormone production or activity.

8. Physiotherapy and Rehabilitative Measures:

• Physical therapy helps patients regain mobility and strength after injuries or procedures, and it can also be beneficial for managing chronic pain conditions.

9. Dietary and Lifestyle Modifications:

• Dietary and lifestyle modifications, including diet adjustments, exercise, and smoking cessation, can play a crucial role in the management and prevention of chronic conditions such as heart disease, diabetes, and obesity.

10. Psychological Counseling and Psychotherapy:

• Mental health disorders such as depression, anxiety, and post-traumatic stress disorder (PTSD) are frequently treated with psychotherapy (talk therapy) and, in some cases, medication.

11. Medical Equipment:

- Using medical devices, such as insulin pumps for diabetes, pacemakers for heart arrhythmias, or prosthetic limbs for amputations, can manage or enhance certain medical conditions.

12. Alternative and Complementary Therapies:

- In addition to conventional treatments, some people utilize complementary and alternative therapies, such as acupuncture, chiropractic therapy, and herbal supplements, to treat their conditions. These should be used with caution and under the supervision of a physician.

13. Hospice care and palliative care:

• Palliative care focuses on improving quality of life and symptom management for patients with severe, life-limiting illnesses. Hospice care provides solace and support at the end of life.

14. Clinical Research:

• Clinical trials entail the evaluation of experimental treatments and therapies for various ailments. Participation in clinical trials can offer access to innovative treatments that are not yet broadly available.

Treatment decisions should always be made in consultation with healthcare professionals who can consider individual factors, including the patient's medical history, preferences, and the specific characteristics of the condition.

The purpose of treatment is to achieve the best feasible outcome while minimizing adverse effects and enhancing the quality of life of the patient.

Experiencing Uterine Cancer

Living with uterine cancer can be a difficult and agonizing journey, but with the right medical care and support, many people are able to manage the disease and maintain a high quality of life. Consider the following factors when coping with uterine cancer:

• Medical treatment is the primary focus in the management of uterine cancer. This may involve surgery, radiation therapy, chemotherapy, hormonal therapy, or a combination thereof. It is essential to collaborate closely with your healthcare team to determine the most appropriate treatment plan for your particular uterine cancer type and stage.

• After initial treatment, it is essential to maintain regular follow-up appointments with your healthcare provider. These appointments are necessary to monitor your progress, detect any indications of recurrence, and manage treatment-related side effects and complications.

• Management of Symptoms Uterine cancer and its treatment can cause a variety of symptoms and adverse effects, including pain, fatigue, nausea, and alterations in bowel or urinary habits. Open communication with your healthcare team is essential for effectively treating these symptoms and enhancing your comfort and quality of life.

• A diagnosis of uterine cancer can elicit a spectrum of emotions, including dread, anxiety, and depression. Seeking emotional support through counseling, support groups, or speaking with a mental health professional can aid in coping with the disease's emotional aspects.

• Supportive Care: Palliative care and symptom management services can provide pain relief and enhance general health. These services aim to improve your quality of life and comfort, regardless of whether you are actively pursuing curative treatment.

• Adopting a healthful lifestyle can have a positive effect on your health and well-being as a whole. This may involve consuming a balanced diet, remaining physically active (if your healthcare provider recommends it), managing tension, and avoiding tobacco and excessive alcohol consumption.

• Fertility and Family Planning: Treatments for uterine cancer, such as hysterectomy, may influence fertility depending on the type and stage of the disease. Before receiving treatment, discuss your fertility preservation options with your healthcare team. In certain circumstances, some women may contemplate fertility-preserving treatments.

• Cancer Survivorship: Many cancer centers offer survivorship programs that offer guidance and resources to help patients transition from active treatment to life after treatment. These programs address cancer survivors' long-term health, emotional well-being, and the challenges they confront.

• Education and Advocacy: Being informed about your condition and treatment options enables you to take an active role in your care. Advocacy organizations and patient support groups can connect you with others who have experienced uterine cancer and provide you with valuable information.

•   Financial and Practical Considerations: Treatment for uterine cancer can be expensive and may hinder your ability to work and manage daily responsibilities. To resolve practical concerns, investigate financial assistance options, disability benefits, and support from social workers or patient advocacy organizations.

Remember that every individual's experience with uterine cancer is unique, and the journey may be distinct for each person. Seeking comprehensive care, establishing a support network, and prioritizing self-care are crucial steps in managing the physical and emotional challenges of uterine cancer and living with it.

CHAPTER FOUR
Survivorship And Post-Treatment Care

Survivorship care is an essential component of cancer management that concentrates on the physical, emotional, and practical needs of individuals who have completed primary cancer treatment and are in remission or are considered cancer survivors.

Follow-up care and ongoing monitoring are essential for the long-term health and well-being of uterine cancer survivors.

Here are some important aspects of uterine cancer survivorship and follow-up care:

• Strategies for Survivorship Care: Many cancer centers offer survivors individualized strategies for survivorship care. These plans detail the patient's diagnosis, treatment history, potential late effects or side effects of treatment, as well as recommendations for follow-up care and screenings. Plans for survivorship care serve as a guide for post-treatment medical care.

• Regular Follow-Up Appointments: Oncologists or gynecologic oncologists typically schedule regular follow-up appointments with uterine cancer survivors. The frequency of these appointments varies based on the specific circumstances of the individual, but they may initially occur every few months and become less frequent over time.

• Physical Examinations: During follow-up appointments, healthcare professionals conduct physical examinations to look for indicators of recurrence or new health problems. They may conduct pelvic examinations and assess the patient's overall health and wellbeing.

• Imaging Studies: Periodic imaging studies, such as ultrasound, CT scans, or MRI, may be prescribed to evaluate the pelvic region and detect any recurrence of cancer or other abnormalities.

• Blood Tests: Blood tests, including cancer markers and routine blood chemistry, may be used to monitor for any changes or indications of recurrence of cancer.

• Survivors should be monitored for potential late effects of cancer treatment, such as alterations in bone density, cardiac function, and hormonal imbalances. Continual management of these concerns may be required.

• As a consequence of cancer treatment, cancer survivors may experience changes in pelvic health, such as vaginal dryness, sexual dysfunction, or urinary issues. Providers of health care can offer guidance and interventions to address these problems.

• Emotional Support: Cancer survivors may continue to face emotional and psychological difficulties resulting from their cancer diagnosis and treatment. Psychosocial support, counseling, and support groups can provide invaluable resources and emotional support.

• Wellness and Lifestyle: Promoting a healthful lifestyle is essential for long-term health. Survivors are often advised to maintain a balanced diet, engage in regular physical activity (if recommended by their healthcare provider), manage tension, and avoid tobacco and excessive alcohol consumption.

• Survivors of uterine cancer can benefit from continued education about their condition, treatment options, and potential long-term effects. Support and advocacy organizations can provide information and opportunities for advocacy and education.

• Some cancer institutions have specialized survivorship clinics or programs that provide comprehensive care and individualized support for cancer survivors.

Healthcare providers are increasingly recognizing the significance of addressing the physical, emotional, and practical aspects of life after cancer treatment.

Survivorship care is an evolving field. Effective survivorship care seeks to improve the quality of life of cancer survivors, promote their well-being, and assist them in resuming a fulfilling and healthy life after cancer treatment.

It is essential for survivors of uterine cancer to maintain open communication with their healthcare team, promptly report any new symptoms or concerns, and actively partake in their follow-up care plan.

Prevention And Danger Minimization

Prevention and risk reduction strategies are essential for reducing the probability of developing uterine cancer and enhancing overall health. Although some risk factors for uterine cancer, such as genetics and age, cannot be altered, there are a number of measures that can be taken to reduce the risk:

• Maintain a Healthy Weight: Obesity is a major risk factor for uterine cancer, as excess adipose tissue can result in elevated estrogen levels. This risk can be reduced by engaging in regular physical activity and maintaining a healthy weight through a balanced diet.

• A diet rich in fruits, vegetables, whole cereals, and lean proteins may reduce the risk of uterine cancer and improve overall health. Additionally, reducing the consumption of high-fat foods and processed meats can be advantageous.

• Regular physical activity not only assists with weight management, but also enhances overall health. As recommended by health guidelines, aim for at least 150 minutes of moderate intensity exercise or 75 minutes of vigorous intensity exercise per week.

• There is an association between heavy alcohol consumption and an increased risk of uterine cancer. If you choose to imbibe, do so in moderation, which for women is one drink per day.

• Quit Smoking: Smoking is linked to several malignancies, including uterine cancer. Cessation of smoking can substantially reduce the risk of cancer and enhance overall health.

• Hormone Replacement Therapy (HRT): Discuss the potential risks and benefits with your healthcare provider if you are contemplating HRT to treat menopause symptoms. Estrogen-only HRT, without progestin, may increase the risk of uterine cancer and should be administered with caution.

• Several studies indicate that the use of oral contraceptives may reduce the risk of uterine cancer. Discuss the use of birth control medications with your healthcare provider, taking your personal medical history into account.

• Routine Health Exams: Routine gynecological examinations and Pap tests can aid in the early detection of any uterine or cervical abnormalities. Follow your doctor's recommendations regarding regular checkups.

• Diabetes and polycystic ovary syndrome (PCOS) are conditions associated with an increased risk of uterine cancer. Managing these conditions effectively through medication and lifestyle modifications can help reduce the risk.

• Genetic Counseling and Testing: If you have a family history of uterine or related malignancies, or inherited cancer syndromes such as Lynch syndrome, you should consider genetic counseling and testing to assess your risk and develop a personalized prevention plan.

• Education and Awareness: It is essential to remain informed about uterine cancer risk factors, symptoms, and warning signs. Knowing one's own risk factors and taking preventive measures and screenings proactively can make a difference.

Despite the fact that these risk reduction strategies can reduce your likelihood of developing uterine cancer, they cannot ensure complete prevention. Regular examinations and early detection are essential components of uterine cancer prevention. Consult a healthcare provider for personalized guidance and risk assessment if you have concerns about your risk factors or symptoms.

Conclusion

Uterine cancer, also known as endometrial cancer, is a major health concern that primarily effects women, particularly those who have gone through menopause. It begins in the uterine lining and can differ in type and stage.

Understanding uterine cancer's risk factors, signs and symptoms, diagnosis, and treatment options is essential for early detection and effective management.

Key learnings include:

• Risk Factors: Several risk factors, such as hormonal imbalances, obesity, age, and familial history, can contribute to the onset of uterine cancer.

• Signs and Symptoms: Abnormal vaginal bleeding is a common symptom, particularly postmenopausal bleeding. Other symptoms may include pelvic pain, discomfort during sexual activity, and a uterus that is enlarged.

• Diagnosis: A combination of medical history, physical exam, imaging studies, biopsies, and laboratory tests are used to confirm the presence and type of uterine cancer through diagnosis.

• Treatment options for uterine cancer include surgery (hysterectomy), radiation therapy, chemotherapy, hormone therapy, and targeted therapy, depending on the cancer's type and stage.

• Survivorship and Follow-Up Care: Survivorship care and regular follow-up appointments are essential for monitoring patients' progress, addressing potential late effects of treatment, and managing symptoms.

• Prevention and Risk Reduction: Modifications to one's lifestyle, such as maintaining a healthy weight, engaging in regular physical activity, and adopting a balanced diet, can assist in lowering the risk of uterine cancer. Regular health examinations, education, and genetic counseling are also essential components of disease prevention.

With medical care, emotional support, and a proactive approach to health, individuals can effectively manage the condition and enhance their quality of life if they have uterine cancer or are uterine cancer survivors.

Remember that individual experiences with uterine cancer can vary, so it is essential to consult with healthcare professionals for individualized guidance and treatment. Early detection, prompt treatment, and a healthy lifestyle are essential for optimizing outcomes and quality of life for uterine cancer patients.

THE END

www.ingramcontent.com/pod-product-compliance
Lightning Source LLC
Chambersburg PA
CBHW072341290526
45794CB00002B/968